Just to say Thank You for Purchasing this Book I want to give you a gift 100% absolutely FREE

A Copy of My Upcoming Book
"*Wheat Belly Decoded*"

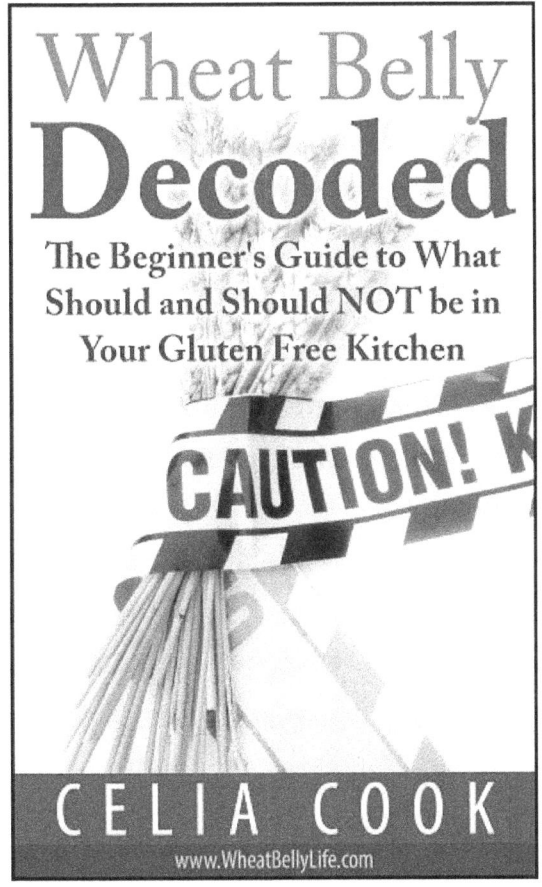

Go to **www.WheatBellyLife.com** to
Reserve Your FREE Copy Now…

Table of Contents

INTRODUCTION   5

EATING GLUTEN-FREE ON THE GO   6

BREAKFAST   7

YUMMY BREAKFAST COOKIES   8
CRUNCHY COTTAGE CHEESE   10
BREAKFAST BURRITOS   11
TRADITIONAL BREAKFAST BURRITOS   12
FRUITY BREAKFAST BURRITOS   13
EGG MUFFINS   14
BREAKFAST QUESADILLAS   15
FROZEN FRUIT SMOOTHIE   16
BREAKFAST GRANOLA   17

LUNCH   18

APPLE SANDWICHES   18
THAI CHICKEN SALAD   19
BENTO BOX WITH EGG SALAD   20
KALE SALAD   22
STRAWBERRY AND SPINACH SALAD   23
BACON AND CHICKEN SANDWICH WITH BLEU CHEESE   24
LUNCH WRAPS WITH PEANUTS, CARROTS, AND SNOW PEAS   26

DINNER   27

CHEESY POTATO BAKE   28
BLACK BEAN BURRITO   29
CHICKEN SATAY   31
TACO IN A BAG   33
HAM AND CHEESE PANINI   34

WHEAT BELLY SNACKS   35

GRANOLA BARS   35
FRUIT SKEWERS   37
BAGEL CHIPS   38
CHEX MIX   39

CONCLUSION   40

Introduction

I want to thank you and congratulate you for purchasing the book, "Gluten-Free To Go: Quick & Easy Gluten-Free Mobile Meals for Your Wheat Belly Life!"

People today are busier than ever, and it can be a challenge to feed your family or even just yourself the good, healthy food needed on a regular basis. When you factor in food sensitivities and allergies, it can feel impossible to eat the kind of food you need without messing up your schedule. Unfortunately, this often means getting stuck in a rut where you eat the same things over and over because they suit your schedule, and you know they are safe.

This is why I pulled together some of my favorite on-the-go recipes. The recipes included here make it easy to get out of that rut and make quick, easy, gluten-free options that can be easily eaten when you are on the run. Since everyone's lives are different, I have included recipes for wheat belly-friendly breakfasts, grab-n-go lunches, mobile-ready dinners, and super portable snacks.

Whether you are looking for breakfast options that you can make in minutes and eat on the train or some yummy snacks that will keep you going through the afternoon slump, this book will get you going with mobile meals that won't upset your wheat belly.

Thanks again for buying this book, I hope you enjoy it!

Celia Cook

Eating Gluten-Free On the Go

For people living a wheat belly life, our fast-paced, always-on-the-go lifestyle can be a big challenge. Trying to find gluten-free foods in fast food restaurants or at convenience stores is almost impossible. This means that you can't rely on being able to find something wheat belly friendly when you are out 'n about. You will need to plan ahead to make sure you can eat no matter where you happen to be at the time.

This means that the first component you need in order to feed your very busy wheat belly is a plan.

The second component is the recipe collection in this book. If you have been eating gluten-free for awhile, you are likely to be familiar with most of the ingredients called for in the recipes included here. If not, never fear, the recipes are easy enough that you will be able to make them without having to get a bunch of things you don't already have in your kitchen.

The third component is the groceries you need to make the delicious recipes in this book. Most of the ingredients used in these recipes should be easy to find in your local grocery store.

The final component for your mobile wheat belly meals is some portable containers you can use to take your delicious wheat belly friendly dishes with you wherever your schedule takes you.

Once you have these components, you will be ready to make all the mobile wheat belly-friendly meals you need to meet the needs of your busy, on-the-go lifestyle.

Breakfast

No matter what your life is like, mornings are likely to be one of the most hectic times of the day. This is why many of the foods marketed for breakfast are ready made like pop-tarts, boxed cereal, and frozen waffles. Unfortunately for us wheat belly folks, the majority of these options are not gluten-free. This means you have to find your own quick ways to ensure you eat this most important meal of the day.

Here are some of my favorite mobile wheat belly breakfast meals. Some of them are things you can make ahead in order to make mornings go more smoothly. Others are super-fast for those mornings that you have nothing made but need to eat fast. My goal was to give you a variety of ideas to help you meet all your wheat belly needs.

Yummy Breakfast Cookies

These yummy cookies can be baked ahead of time so you have a great breakfast option ready to go. I like to bake up a batch on Sunday afternoon so that I have them throughout the week. This recipe will make you about 8 cookies.

<u>*Ingredients:*</u>

- 1 ¼ cups all-purpose, gluten-free flour
- ½ teaspoon baking soda
- 1 tablespoon ground cinnamon
- 1 teaspoon ground nutmeg
- ¼ teaspoon salt
- 2 tablespoons butter
- ¼ cup vegetable oil
- ¼ cup dark brown sugar
- 3 tablespoons granulated white sugar
- 1 egg
- ¼ cup carrot puree
- 1 teaspoon vanilla extract
- ½ cup gluten-free oats
- ½ cup gluten-free flake cereal
- 1/3 cup raisins
- ¼ cup of dried berries
- 1/3 cup chopped nuts

<u>*Directions:*</u>

Pre-heat oven to 350°F.

Combine first five ingredients in a medium mixing bowl, and mix using a whisk. In a separate bowl, add butter, oil, and both kinds of sugar. Use a mixer on high to combine these ingredients until the sugar has been fully incorporated. Add the egg, carrot puree, and vanilla to the butter mixture, and mix on high for about 30 seconds. Slowly add the flour mixture from the first bowl into the wet ingredients, mixing as you add. Once the flour mixture is mixed into the wet ingredients, add the oats, cereal, raisins, berries, and nuts. Use the mixer on low speed to combine everything.

Scoop the batter into balls on a cookie sheet, and then flatten with a big spoon. Bake for about 12 minutes, and then cool completely on a rack before storing.

Crunchy Cottage Cheese

This easy breakfast option can be assembled ahead of time and stored in the fridge, but it can also be easily assembled as needed, even on the busiest mornings. As an added bonus, it also makes a great snack. This makes a single serving.

Ingredients:

- ½ cup of cottage cheese
- ½ cup of your favorite gluten free cereal
- ½ cup of canned fruit, drained

Directions:

Add all three ingredients to a bowl and stir to combine.

Variables

Like I said, you can make this ahead of time, but if you do, keep the cereal packaged separately until you are ready to eat it, otherwise it will get soggy.

You can use whichever kind of cottage cheese you like best. I like 1%, but if you prefer fat free, use that instead.

Canned fruit that I have found that works well with this recipe includes peaches, pears, and mandarin oranges, but feel free to experiment and try any kind of fruit you love.

You can also use fresh fruit with this recipe, like chopped bananas or any kind of berries. Using fresh fruit will generally take a little longer.

Breakfast Burritos

Breakfast burritos have become very popular in recent years, and you can find them on almost every fast food restaurant's breakfast menu. Unfortunately, they are generally made with flour tortillas and may include sausage, ham, or egg products that have gluten added to them. However, you can make them at home if you have a couple minutes and the right wheat belly ingredients.

You can use pre-made, gluten-free tortillas which are now available in most grocery stores, or you can use the recipe from my Wheat Belly Bread book for gluten-free crepes. Here are a couple different ways to make this great grab-n-go breakfast.

Traditional Breakfast Burritos

If you are lamenting the loss of the breakfast burrito from your favorite fast food place, this recipe will make things right. Not only will it give you the flavors you crave without upsetting your belly, it will taste even better than the ones you remember. This makes 4 burritos.

Ingredients:

- 2 teaspoons vegetable oil
- 8 ounces pre-cooked gluten-free sausage, chopped up
- 1 cup frozen hash browns (check the label to make sure they are gluten-free), defrosted
- ¼ cup chopped onions
- ¼ cup chopped green peppers
- 8 large eggs
- 4 gluten-free tortillas or 8 gluten-free crepes
- 1 avocado, sliced
- ½ cup finely shredded cheddar cheese
- 2 tablespoons salsa

Directions:

In a non-stick skillet, use the oil to sauté the onions and peppers for about 5 minutes. Add the sausage and potatoes; continue sautéing for about 10 minutes. Crack the eggs into a bowl and whisk until they are well scrambled. Pour the eggs over the sausage and potato mixture and cook, stirring, until the eggs set.

Heat the tortillas or crepes in the microwave. Assemble burritos using the egg, potato, and sausage mixture, a slice of avocado, cheese, and salsa. Wrap in aluminum foil if you are taking it with you.

Fruity Breakfast Burritos

For a completely different take on the breakfast burrito, try this tasty recipe. While you can use gluten-free tortillas for this recipe as well, I like it better with the gluten-free crepes. This makes 10 small burritos.

Ingredients:

- ½ cup white sugar
- 1 tablespoon ground cinnamon
- Spray butter
- 10 gluten-free crepes
- 1 ¼ cups yogurt (vanilla or your favorite flavor)
- ½ pint blueberries
- ½ pint raspberries

Directions:

Combine the sugar and cinnamon in a small bowl, and then sprinkle some over the surface of a plate that is larger than your crepes.

Do the following for each crepe. Spray one side of the crepe with spray butter, and then put the crepe butter side down on the plate with the cinnamon sugar. Spread yogurt over the tortilla, and lay a row of fruit down the middle of the crepe, and roll the crepe around the fruit. Move the "burrito" to a clean plate and sprinkle more cinnamon sugar on the plate before repeating.

Egg Muffins

If you are missing your morning muffin, this yummy alternative will get your day started with a punch of protein instead of all those carbs. You can make these ahead and keep them in the fridge to eat over the course of the week.

Ingredients:

- 8 ounces of sausage, removed from casing
- ¼ cup diced green bell pepper
- ¼ cup chopped onions
- 1 tablespoon of olive oil
- 3 tablespoons fresh chopped basil
- ½ cup chopped spinach
- ¼ cup chopped tomatoes
- 10 eggs
- Salt and pepper to taste

Directions:

Preheat the oven to 375°F, and use cooking spray to prep a muffin pan.

Cook the sausage, onions, and peppers in a skillet with the olive oil until the sausage is cooked through. Crack all the eggs into a bowl, and scramble with a fork. Add the sausage mixture, spinach, tomatoes, and basil, and stir to combine.

Fill muffin cups about ¾ of the way full and bake for 25-30 minutes. Muffins are done when the egg has set in the middle of the muffins.

Breakfast Quesadillas

Quesadillas always make great breakfast options that you can eat on the move. Using corn tortillas allows you to get the same quesadilla feel without the gluten. This makes 2 servings.

<u>Ingredients:</u>

- 6 slices of bacon
- 4 eggs
- Salt and pepper to taste
- 4 corn tortillas
- 1 cup shredded Colby jack cheese
- Cooking spray
- Salsa

<u>Directions:</u>

Cook bacon in the microwave. Drain grease, and chop into small pieces.

Crack eggs in a bowl, scramble with a fork, and season with salt and pepper. Cook the eggs in a skillet pan until set.

Place a tortilla on your plate, and sprinkle with cheese. Add half the bacon and half the eggs. Sprinkle more cheese over the bacon and eggs. Cover with another tortilla. Heat the quesadilla in the microwave for 1 minute in order to melt the cheese. Spray a clean skillet with cooking spray, and put the quesadilla in for a minute on each side. Repeat with the other two tortillas. Cut into wedges to eat with salsa on the side.

Frozen Fruit Smoothie

Smoothies from the shop down the street have gotten a bad rap, but that doesn't mean that all smoothies are bad for you. A smoothie with the right ingredients can be a great gluten-free breakfast. This makes one smoothie.

Ingredients:

- 3 cups frozen berries or fruit
- ½ cup apple juice
- ½ cup water
- ½ cup yogurt
- 2 tablespoons of flax or chia seeds
- 1 teaspoon agave syrup

Directions:

Combine all ingredients in the blender and blend until smooth.

Breakfast Granola

The ultimate in grab-n-go, this granola can be made ahead and stored in easy-to-grab batches. Since it doesn't require utensils or even a bowl, you can grab a bag of this delicious gluten-free granola and eat it on the road, on the train, or wherever you are going on the busiest of mornings.

Ingredients:

- 1/3 cup orange juice
- 1/3 cup honey
- ¼ cup packed brown sugar
- 2 teaspoons vegetable oil
- 1 teaspoon vanilla extract
- 2 cups gluten-free steel cut oats
- 1/3 cup ground flaxseed
- ½ cup chopped nuts
- 2 teaspoons ground cinnamon
- 1/3 cup dried cranberries
- Cooking spray

Directions:

Preheat your oven to 300°F. In a small sauce pan, heat the orange juice, honey, and brown sugar over medium heat. Stir frequently until the sugar has completely dissolved. Remove from heat. Add oil and vanilla.

Combine oats, flaxseed, nuts, cinnamon, and cranberries in a medium bowl. Pour honey mixture over oat mixture, and stir to combine. Spray a cookie sheet with cooking spray, and spread the granola mixture over the pan. Bake for 10 minutes, stirring occasionally. Return to the oven for an additional 10 minutes. Remove from the oven, and scoop into a bowl. Allow to cool, and store in a plastic bag.

Lunch

For those of us living a wheat belly life, lunch can be one of the hardest meals of the day because it is the one we are least likely to be eating at home. The easiest way to make sure you have a great gluten-free lunch is to bring your own from home. These lunch ideas can be packed up and taken with you wherever your busy life leads you.

Apple Sandwiches

You may not be able to eat regular bread, but that doesn't mean you can't have delicious sandwiches for lunch. One great way to do this is with slices of apple instead of slices of bread. If you are making these ahead, drop the apple slices in a mixture of lemon juice and water for a few minutes before assembling your sandwich to keep the slices from turning brown.

Ingredients:

- 1 apple, cored and sliced into rings
- Peanut or almond butter
- Gluten-free granola
- Raisins

Directions:

Use the apple slices like bread, spread the peanut butter over the slice, sprinkle with granola and raisins, and top with another apple slice.

Thai Chicken Salad

Not being able to eat gluten doesn't mean you have to settle for boring or tasteless fare, and this tasty chicken salad will definitely help spice up your lunch hour. You can also use this salad as filling for lettuce wraps or to top a salad of leafy greens. This makes 4 servings.

Ingredients:

- 3 large cucumbers
- 1 tablespoon salt
- ½ cup white sugar
- ½ cup rice wine vinegar
- 2 jalapeno peppers
- ¼ cup cilantro
- ½ cup peanuts
- 1 can of cooked chicken

Directions:

Peel the cucumbers, and cut them in half lengthwise. Cut off the seeded part in the middle, and cut the remaining parts into thin slices. Put the cucumbers in a colander, and sprinkle with salt. Let this set in the sink while you prep the other ingredients.

In a medium-sized bowl, combine the sugar and vinegar. Whisk until the sugar has dissolved. Seed and chop the jalapeños, and add them to the vinegar mixture. Rinse the cucumbers with cold water, and shake to remove as much water as possible. Add to the vinegar mixture. Chop the cilantro and the peanuts, and add those as well. Chop the canned chicken into small bites, and add to the mixture. Stir to combine all ingredients.

Bento Box with Egg Salad

Traditionally, a bento box is a single-portion meal packed in a special box. Using this concept, we can make fantastically flavorful wheat belly lunches filled with delicious foods that we will look forward to eating. This makes 1 serving.

Ingredients:

- 2 eggs
- 2 tablespoons celery, diced
- 1 tablespoon mayonnaise
- 2 teaspoons Dijon mustard
- 1 teaspoon minced onions
- 2 large lettuce leaves
- ½ cup berries
- ½ cup banana slices
- 2 tablespoons vanilla yogurt
- 2/3 cup broccoli florets
- 6 cherry tomatoes
- 5 gluten-free crackers
- 10 unsalted cashews
- 1 tablespoon bittersweet chocolate chips

Directions:

Hard boil the eggs. Once they are cool, peel and chop the eggs. Combine eggs, mayo, mustard, and onions in a bowl, and mash together to break up the egg and mix together. Line one container with the lettuce leaves, and scoop the egg salad onto the lettuce leaves.

In another container, mix the yogurt, berries, and banana together. Place the broccoli and tomatoes in another container and the crackers in their own container. Lastly, combine the cashews and chocolate chips in their own container for a sweet, delicious dessert.

Kale Salad

Kale is the super food of the moment with good reason. It is packed with nutritional value and boosts the flavor and texture of any salad it is added into. Eating for your wheat belly doesn't always mean eating things that usually contain gluten. It also means choosing things that are naturally gluten free. This fantastic salad is a great example of a tasty lunch that doesn't require any changes to meet your wheat belly needs. This makes one serving.

Ingredients:

- 3 tablespoons lemon juice
- 2 tablespoons olive oil
- Salt and pepper to taste
- 1 bunch kale
- ¼ cup dates or other dried fruit
- 1 apple
- ¼ cup nuts, chopped
- ¼ cup parmesan cheese, finely grated

Directions:

Wash the kale, remove the ribs, and slice the leaves into thin strips. In a bowl large enough to hold all the kale, combine the lemon juice, olive oil, salt, and pepper. Whisk together until well combined. Add the sliced kale, and use tongs to toss until kale is coated. Set aside.

Slice the dates or other dried fruit into thin slivers. Peel and core the apple, and then chop it into thin matchsticks. Add dried fruit, nuts, and cheese to the bowl with the kale. Toss with tongs to combine and serve.

Strawberry and Spinach Salad

This is another great, naturally gluten-free salad that will provide you with a delicious lunch that is easy to make, easy to pack up, and easy to eat just about anywhere. This makes one serving.

Ingredients:

- 1 cup strawberries
- 2 tablespoons white wine vinegar
- 2 tablespoons fresh basil leaves
- 1 tablespoon olive oil
- 1 teaspoon sugar
- Kosher salt and freshly ground black pepper
- 2 cups baby Spinach
- ¼ cup feta cheese

Directions:

Remove the tops of the strawberries, and cut them into thin slices. Finely chop the basil. Add half the strawberries, chopped basil, vinegar, oil, sugar, salt, and pepper to your blender. Blend until smooth. Set dressing aside.

Wash and dry the spinach, removing stems if necessary. Combine spinach, remaining strawberries, and cheese to a large bowl. Add dressing, and toss to coat before serving.

Bacon and Chicken Sandwich with Bleu Cheese

If you are looking for something a little more substantial for lunch than one of those tasty salads, this sandwich may be just what you need. You can use any store-bought, gluten-free bread, but I like this recipe best with a homemade Dark Sandwich Bread made with Teff. You can find the recipe for this bread in my Wheat Belly Bread book. This makes four sandwiches.

Ingredients:

- 4 slices bacon, thickly sliced
- ¼ cup mayonnaise
- 2 teaspoons Worcestershire sauce
- 1 teaspoon Dijon mustard
- 1 garlic clove, minced
- 8 slices gluten-free bread
- ¼ cup soft blue cheese
- 4 leaves romaine lettuce
- 6 ounces of cooked chicken, sliced
- 4 ounces roasted red peppers
- ½ avocado

Directions:

Cook bacon, and cut each slice in half. In a small bowl, combine mayonnaise, Worcestershire sauce, mustard, and garlic. Whisk together until well combined. Slice avocado into thin slices. Toast the slices of bread.

To assemble each sandwich, spread the mayonnaise mixture on one piece or bread. Spread the bleu cheese on the other slice of bread. Place one lettuce leaf on the bottom slice of bread. Then layer a quarter of the chicken, a quarter of the red peppers, a quarter of the avocado, and two pieces of bacon. Top with the other piece of bread.

Lunch Wraps with Peanuts, Carrots, and Snow Peas

One of the things I missed the most when I decided to go gluten-free was the lunch wraps I used to eat almost every day. Fortunately, as more and more people opted for a gluten-free life, the variety of gluten-free food available at my local grocery store increased, including several different kinds of gluten-free tortillas. These can be used to make your favorite wraps. Keep in mind that these tortillas, like many gluten-free foods, don't taste exactly the same as the flour tortillas you are used to using. There are several different kinds of tortillas available in many stores that are made with different ingredients. Try a couple until you find one you like the best. Then fill it with your favorite filling. Here is mine. This makes 2 servings.

Ingredients:

- ¼ cup crunchy peanut butter
- 1 teaspoon gluten-free Asian chili paste
- 1 tablespoon gluten-free soy sauce
- 2 tablespoons water
- 2 gluten-free tortillas
- 1 cup carrots
- 1 cup snap peas

Directions:

Combine the first four ingredients in a small bowl. Whisk together until well combined. Finely shred the carrots, and slice the snow peas into diagonal pieces. Spread half the peanut butter mixture down the middle of each tortilla. Add half the carrots and snow peas. Roll the tortilla up, wrap-style. Wrap in plastic or aluminum foil to store for lunch.

Dinner

Traditionally, dinner is the easiest meal of the day to make in a wheat belly-friendly way, but with today's busy schedules, this isn't always the case. Some of the recipes in this section are simple to take with you wherever you have to go, while others are quick and easy for families on the go. Whether you are eating on the go because you are working late or need to feed hungry kids after soccer practice, these dinner recipes will satisfy your wheat belly needs and your busy schedule.

Cheesy Potato Bake

This tasty dinner can be made ahead of time and packaged into easy-to-reheat-and-eat containers. It is filled with cheesy goodness that everyone in your family will love. This makes 12 servings.

Ingredients:

- 4 pounds potatoes
- Cooking spray
- 2 teaspoons chili powder
- 2 teaspoons garlic powder
- Salt and pepper to taste
- 6 tablespoons butter, cubed
- 8 ounces shredded Cheddar cheese
- 1 bottle Ranch dressing

Directions:

Preheat oven to 400°F. Chop potatoes into ¼ inch cubes and place them in a 9" x 13" baking dish coated with cooking spray. Sprinkle chili powder and garlic powder over the potatoes. Season potatoes with salt and pepper to taste. Distribute butter throughout the dish of potatoes. Cover dish with foil and bake for 1 hour. Remove from oven, and mix in cheese and ranch dressing. Return to oven, uncovered, and cook for 10-15 more minutes until the cheese is melted and bubbly.

Black Bean Burrito

Burritos are a great mobile dinner that is always a family favorite, but without some modifications, burritos just aren't suitable to a wheat belly life. Most traditional seasoning mixes contain ingredients that are not wheat belly-friendly, and the tortillas generally used for burritos are made with flour. However, you can still make super-mobile burritos packed with delicious southwest flavors by using gluten-free tortillas (like those used for the lunch wraps) and individual spices instead of a pre-packaged mix. This makes 6 burritos.

Ingredients:

- 1 15 ½ ounce can of black beans
- 2 teaspoons chili powder
- 1 teaspoon ground cumin
- 1 teaspoon garlic powder
- 1 teaspoon onion powder
- 1 cup instant whole grain brown rice
- Water
- 1 ½ cups salsa
- 1 cup shredded Colby Jack cheese
- 6 gluten-free tortillas
- 6 tablespoons sour cream

Directions:

Rinse and drain beans, and pour into a large saucepan. Add spices and stir to combine with beans. Add uncooked rice and the amount of water required per the instructions on the rice package. Bring to a boil, cover, and reduce heat. Simmer for about 10 minutes (refer to the directions on the rice package for exact timing) until rice is done.

Add 2/3 cup of the salsa to the rice and beans, and stir to combine.

Assemble the burritos by warming the tortillas in the microwave for 15-30 seconds before sprinkling cheese down the middle of a tortilla. Then spoon about a half a cup of the beans and rice over the cheese before rolling up. Top with a spoon of salsa and a spoon of sour cream. For a more mobile version, wrap the burrito in foil, and either add the sour cream and salsa to the burrito before it is rolled up, or bring the sour cream and salsa in small containers and use like dipping sauces.

Chicken Satay

Is there anything more mobile than meat on a stick? This delicious dish is sure to become a favorite for those on the go. Make these tasty skewers up ahead of time for a fast wheat belly-friendly dinner that you won't even need a fork to enjoy. This makes 5 servings of 2 skewers each.

Ingredients:

For Marinade

- ½ cup coconut milk
- 1 clove garlic, minced
- 1 teaspoon curry powder
- 1 ½ teaspoons brown sugar
- ½ teaspoon salt
- ½ teaspoon ground black pepper

For Chicken

- 1   pound boneless chicken breast
- 10 (6 inch) wooden skewers, or as needed, soaked in water for 30 minutes

For Sauce

- 1 cup coconut milk
- 1 tablespoon curry powder
- ½ cup creamy peanut butter
- ¾ cup chicken stock
- ¼ cup brown sugar
- 2 tablespoons lime or lemon juice
- 1 teaspoon soy sauce
- Salt to taste'

Directions:

In a plastic bag large enough to hold the chicken, combine the ingredients for the sauce. Seal the bag, and shake to combine. Remove skin from chicken, if necessary, and slice into 1 inch strips. Add to marinade bag, and place in the refrigerator for at least 2 hours. Soak the skewers in water for about 30 minutes before cooking the chicken.

To make the sauce, combine all sauce ingredients except the soy sauce in a medium sauce pan. Heat sauce to a simmer over medium to high heat, and stir constantly for about 5 minutes. The sauce will be smooth and thick when it is done. Add the soy sauce, and stir to combine.

When you are ready to cook, preheat the grill. Remove the chicken from the marinade, and slide onto the skewers. Cook on the grill for about 5 minutes per side until done. Serve with warm sauce.

Taco in a Bag

This recipe might seem a little strange, but it you are looking for a fun, wheat belly-friendly way to eat on the go, you can't beat the taco in a bag. Because Fritos corn chips are naturally gluten-free, this recipe is great for any wheat belly life. Just make sure you use a taco seasoning mix that is gluten-free. This makes 4 servings.

Ingredients:

- 1 pound lean ground beef
- 1 package gluten-free taco seasoning mix
- 4 small bags Fritos corn chips
- 2 cups lettuce, shredded
- 1 medium tomato, diced
- 1 cup cheddar cheese, shredded
- 1/3 cup salsa
- ½ cup sour cream
- 1/3 cup guacamole

Directions:

In a large skillet, brown the ground beef, and then follow the directions on the taco seasoning mix. While the meat is cooking, gently crush the corn chips in the unopened bags to break them into smaller pieces. Then clip one corner of the bag, and use scissors to slit the bag open along the longer side edge. Once the meat is cooked, let it cool for about 5 minutes and then add a quarter of itto each bag. Then add a quarter of each of the other ingredients to each bag and serve. This can easily be eaten with chilled meat, which makes it ideal for on the go eating. All you need is the pre-made ingredients, the bags of chips, and a couple forks.

Ham and Cheese Panini

Panini's can make great mobile meals. Since you can fill them with just about anything, you can be sure that you can make a dinner everyone will love. While you can make them without a sandwich grill, the signature ridges of the Panini are easier to make with a sandwich grill like the George Foreman model sold in most stores. To make a wheat belly-friendly Panini, use the sourdough bread recipe in my Wheat Belly bread book. The recipe here is fairly simple, but you can use whatever fillings you like best. This makes one serving.

Ingredients:

- Olive oil
- 2 pieces gluten-free sourdough bread
- 1 cup chopped ham
- 1 cup shredded cheddar cheese

Directions:

Preheat the sandwich grill. Brush one side of the sourdough slices with olive oil. Place one slice, oil side down on the preheated grill. Layer the ham and cheese on the bread, and top with the other slice of bread, oil side up. Lower the top of the sandwich grill, and cook for 3-5 minutes. Sandwich is ready when the signature ridges are clearly formed, and the cheese is melted.

Wheat Belly Snacks

Snacking can be very challenging for those living a wheat belly life. Your best bet is to pack snacks from home since it isn't always easy to find gluten-free snacks at gas stations or in convenience stores. These snacks are easy to make, easy to pack up, and easy to eat on the go.

Granola Bars

Most commercial granola bars have hidden or not so hidden gluten-filled ingredients, which mean they aren't a good fit for wheat belly folks. However, this doesn't mean you can't enjoy this healthy, mobile snack, it just means you have to make them yourself. Make sure you get quick-cooking oats and chocolate chips that are gluten-free, as not all options in the stores are made without gluten. This makes 24 individual granola bars.

Ingredients:

- Cooking spray
- 3 cups gluten-free quick-cooking oats
- 1 can sweetened condensed milk
- 2 tablespoons butter, melted
- 1 cup coconut, finely flaked
- 1 cup nuts, chopped
- 1 cup gluten-free miniature semisweet chocolate chips
- ½ cup sweetened dried cranberries or other dried fruit

Directions:

Preheat your oven to 350°F. Coat a 9" x 13" inch baking pan with cooking spray.

In a large bowl, combine oats, condensed milk, butter, coconut, nuts, chocolate chips, and dried fruit. Mix all ingredients together by hand until well combined. Move mixture into the baking pan, and press flat. Bake for 20-30 minutes, depending on how chewy/crunchy you want your granola bars to be. Remove from the oven, and allow to cool for 5-10 minutes. Cut into squares, and remove from the pan. Cool completely before wrapping in plastic wrap to store.

Fruit Skewers

Food on a stick makes a great snack too, and these fruit skewers are easy to make and easy to eat. They are perfect for on-the-go families and busy professionals who crave something sweet but who don't want to risk gluten exposure with a sweet treat from a store. This makes 5 servings of 2 skewers each.

<u>Ingredients:</u>

- 5 large strawberries
- ¼ cantaloupe
- 2 bananas
- 2 apples
- 40 blueberries or blackberries
- 10 skewers

<u>Directions:</u>

Wash all fruit. Remove the top of each strawberry, and slice the strawberry in half. Cut the cantaloupe into cubes, and peel the bananas before cutting them into chunks. Chop the apple into chunks.

Thread each skewer with a strawberry, a blueberry, a cube of cantaloupe, a blueberry, a chunk of banana, a blueberry, a chunk of apple, and a blueberry.

Bagel Chips

When you are craving something crunchy, bagel chips can provide a healthier option to chips, but it isn't always easy to find gluten-free bagel chips. You can use the recipe for bagels in my Wheat Belly Bread book to make bagels, and then use this recipe to turn them into chips.

Ingredients:

- 3 tablespoons butter
- 2 cloves garlic, chopped
- 5 stale plain gluten-free bagels
- ½ cup parmesan cheese, grated

Directions:

Preheat oven to 325°F. In a small saucepan, add the butter and the garlic, and heat until the butter is melted. Cut the bagels into thin slices. Brush one side of each bagel slice with the garlic butter, and place it on a cookie sheet covered with aluminum foil. Once the pan is full of chips, sprinkle the chips with the cheese.

Bake for 10 minutes. Remove pan from the oven, and flip each chip over. Brush the other side with garlic butter, and sprinkle the chips with cheese. Bake for 10 more minutes. Remove, and allow to cool completely before storing in an air tight container.

Chex Mix

Thankfully, many of the cereals made by Chex® are naturally gluten-free and always have been. This means you can still make this tasty snack with only minor modifications. Because most of the Chex® Mix versions sold in stores contain pretzels and other ingredients that contain gluten, you are better off making it yourself. This makes about 18 servings.

Ingredients:

- 4 cups Corn Chex® cereal
- 4 cups Rice Chex® cereal
- 1 cup nuts
- 1 cup gluten-free bagel chips, broken into 1-inch pieces
- 6 tablespoons butter
- 2 tablespoons Worcestershire sauce
- 1 ½ teaspoons salt
- ¾ teaspoon garlic powder
- ½ teaspoon onion powder

Directions:

Preheat oven to 250°F. In a large bowl, combine cereal, nuts, and bagel chips. Melt butter. Add Worcestershire sauce and spices to the melted butter. Pour slowly over the cereal mixture, stirring to coat. Move mixture to a 9" x 13" baking pan, and place in the oven. Bake for 1 hour, stirring every 15 minutes until done.

Remove from oven, and spread mixture out over cool baking sheets covered with paper towels, and allow to cool completely. Store in an airtight container.

Conclusion

Thank you again for purchasing this book!

I hope this book gave you some great ideas for how to meet the needs of your busy schedule and your wheat belly!

With the recipes in this book, you have a variety of options for all three daily meals which will make it easier than ever to make sure you always have a grab-n-go option that won't make you sick.

Once you start making mobile wheat belly meals, feel free to experiment. Try different types of gluten-free tortillas, gluten-free breads, and even making your own gluten-free bread options.

Finally, if you enjoyed this book, please take the time to share your thoughts and post a review on Amazon. It'd be greatly appreciated!

Thank you and good luck!

Celia Cook

www.ingramcontent.com/pod-product-compliance
Lightning Source LLC
Chambersburg PA
CBHW070510290526
45790CB00003B/1175